FAMILY FIRST AID

FAMILY FIRST AID

Margaret Barca

CLAREMONT BOOKS

PENGUIN BOOKS

Published by the Penguin Group
Penguin Books Ltd, 27 Wrights Lane, London W8 5TZ, England
Penguin Books USA Inc., 375 Hudson Street, New York, New York 10014, USA
Penguin Books Australia Ltd, Ringwood, Victoria, Australia
Penguin Books Canada Ltd, 10 Alcorn Avenue, Toronto, Ontario, Canada M4V 3B2
Penguin Books (NZ) Ltd, 182–190 Wairau Road, Auckland 10, New Zealand

Penguin Books Ltd, Registered Offices: Harmondsworth, Middlesex, England

First published by Penguin Books 1991

This edition published by Claremont Books,
an imprint of Godfrey Cave Associates Limited,
42 Bloomsbury Street, London WC1B 3QJ,
under licence from Penguin Books Ltd, 1995

ISBN 1 85471 761 8

CONTENTS

vi • Contents

ACKNOWLEDGEMENTS

In the course of preparing *Family First Aid* we received considerable help and advice from a number of medical organisations. We would particularly like to thank Ella Tyler, Deputy Chairman of the Australian Resuscitation Council, for her meticulous reading of the manuscript and her comprehensive and invaluable suggestions. Alison Verhoeven, National Training Officer of St John Ambulance Australia, also kindly gave the manuscript a close reading.

We are very grateful to Dr D. R. Gauld of the Asthma Foundation of Victoria, Christine Lyons of the Diabetes Foundation of Victoria, Jenny Murray of the Epilepsy Foundation of Victoria and Dr Frank Oberklaid of the Department of Ambulatory Paediatrics, Royal Children's Hospital, Victoria, for their detailed information and critical comments in specialised areas of family medicine.

We would also like to thank Dr Michael Apple for adapting the UK edition.

EMERGENCY PHONE NUMBERS

Fill in the phone numbers for the following services and keep them up to date. In an emergency they could help save someone's life.

Ambulance _____

Children's hospital _____

Dental emergency service _____

Doctor _____

Electricity emergency service _____

Fire brigade _____

Police _____

In a life-threatening emergency dial 999 for police, ambulance and fire brigade.

INTRODUCTION

First aid is just that – the immediate attention and treatment given when someone suffers an injury or sudden illness. In some cases the injury or illness will be minor, and common sense and basic treatment will be all that are needed. Never forget that staying calm and being sympathetic and reassuring are part of the treatment, even for minor childhood cuts and grazes.

There are, however, accidents and illnesses that are serious, even life-threatening. In these cases you have only a few minutes in which to act to prevent permanent disability, brain damage or even death.

The life-saving techniques of artificial respiration (AR) and cardiopulmonary resuscitation (CPR) are explained at the beginning of this book, but it is vital that you study these procedures under a qualified instructor, using an approved resuscitation training manikin. Resuscitation techniques can be mastered by everyone, but they are skills for which practice is essential. If you've practised with an expert instructor you will be able to act instantly, confidently and effectively in an emergency, and this may well mean the difference between life and death for the casualty.

Accidents *can* be prevented. Because so many accidents occur in the home, we have included a chapter on family safety so that you can make your home safer. And because of the frequency of road accidents, we have also included information on what to do at the scene of a traffic accident. But, once again, prevent accidents, by, for example, obeying the speed and alcohol limitations and driving safely. You could save your own life, as well as someone else's.

HOW TO USE THIS BOOK

Family First Aid is designed to be as simple and accessible as possible. You will find that the step-by-step instructions throughout and the A to Z listing of accidents and sudden illnesses in the second section make it easy to follow, even in an emergency.

The first section of the book (Emergency, First Aid and Safety Procedures) provides essential information on treating medical emergencies, such as unconsciousness, absence of breathing and blood circulation failure. A chapter on ROAD TRAFFIC ACCIDENTS is included in this section. The first part of the book also offers information on FAMILY SAFETY and on the articles you should have at hand in case of accidents or sudden illnesses and how to apply these (see FIRST AID KITS; DRESSINGS, PADS AND BANDAGES; SLINGS; SPLINTS). You should read the first section now so that you know where to find essential information in an emergency and to familiarise yourself with first aid procedures.

The second section of the book (A to Z of Injuries and Illnesses) provides chapters, organised alphabetically for easy reference, on the most common major and minor sudden medical occurrences that you may have to deal with.

Cross-references within a chapter to other, relevant chapters, in either section of the book, are given in SMALL CAPITAL LETTERS.

EMERGENCY, FIRST AID AND SAFETY PROCEDURES

WHAT TO DO BEFORE
AN EMERGENCY

- Read carefully all the information on first aid techniques given in this book, *now*, before an accident or sudden serious illness occurs. Don't wait for an emergency.
- Learn how to apply artificial respiration (AR) and cardiopulmonary resuscitation (CPR) (see EMERGENCY TECHNIQUES): they are life-saving techniques. It is essential to practise with a trained instructor because only practice will give you the confidence and ability to act instantly and correctly in the vital few minutes that can mean the difference between life and death. The St John Ambulance and the Red Cross, for example, run first aid courses.
- Make sure you have a well-equipped first aid kit at home, in the car and boat, and on holidays (see FIRST AID KITS).

EMERGENCY PRIORITIES

A person's life is in danger if he or she is unconscious. The airway may be blocked, breathing may have stopped and blood circulation may have ceased.

You need to:

- act immediately because brain damage or death can quickly result
- carry out the procedures outlined in the chart on page 5, in the order given
- follow the instructions given in the next chapter, EMERGENCY TECHNIQUES, for each of the procedures mentioned in the chart on page 5.

Remember in an Emergency

- **Do not** approach a casualty unless it is safe to do so. Check whether there is any danger for you, others or the injured person first.
- Even though you will feel upset, it's important to act as calmly as possible and to reassure any casualties.
- Every minute is vital.
- **Do not** move a casualty unless it is absolutely essential for safety (see MOVING A CASUALTY).
- **Do not** leave a casualty alone. Send someone else for medical aid immediately. However, if you are the only person present in an emergency and help is unlikely

to arrive you will have to go for aid yourself as soon as possible. Dial 999.

- Messages given to emergency services should be brief: indicate place, nature of the emergency, number of people involved and nature and extent of injuries or illness.
- Do not give anything to eat or drink.

See also ROAD TRAFFIC ACCIDENTS.

Action

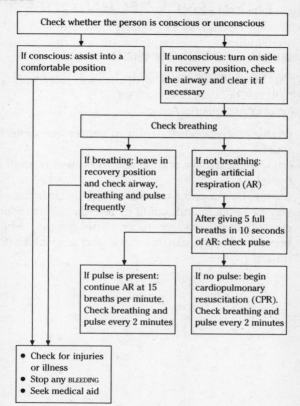

Check whether the person is conscious or unconscious

If conscious: assist into a comfortable position

If unconscious: turn on side in recovery position, check the airway and clear it if necessary

Check breathing

If breathing: leave in recovery position and check airway, breathing and pulse frequently

If not breathing: begin artificial respiration (AR)

After giving 5 full breaths in 10 seconds of AR: check pulse

If pulse is present: continue AR at 15 breaths per minute. Check breathing and pulse every 2 minutes

If no pulse: begin cardiopulmonary resuscitation (CPR). Check breathing and pulse every 2 minutes

- Check for injuries or illness
- Stop any BLEEDING
- Seek medical aid

EMERGENCY TECHNIQUES

CHECKING FOR UNCONSCIOUSNESS

When the normal activity of the brain is interrupted, a person can become unconscious.

An unconscious person is:

- unable to respond normally to simple questions or touch
- unaware of danger and unable to protect himself or herself
- unable, by coughing or swallowing, to clear the airway of saliva, blood, vomit or foreign matter, which can obstruct the air tubes. The tongue, which becomes floppy, can fall back and also block the throat.

Action

1 Assess whether the person is unconscious by asking simple questions or giving simple commands, such as 'What is your name?' or 'Open your eyes', and gently shaking him or her by the shoulders. If there is no response the person is unconscious.

2 Place the casualty in the recovery position (see box, pp. 8–9) and check the airway, breathing and pulse (see below).

3 If the unconscious person is breathing and has a pulse, maintain him or her in the recovery position, ensuring the airway remains clear and open and frequently checking breathing and pulse until medical aid arrives.

RECOVERY POSITION

1 Kneel beside the casualty, facing their chest.
2 Turn their head towards you and raise the chin to maintain the airway.
3 Place their hand nearest to you under their buttock and the other arm across the chest.

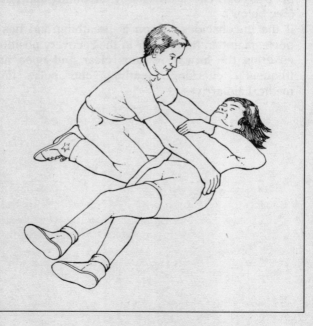

4 Position their upper arm at right angles across their chest so it can act as a support.

5 Hold the hip or the clothes on the far side and carefully pull the body over towards you.

6 Bend the upper leg at right angles to their hip to provide greater support.

7 Make sure that the chin is raised to maintain the airway.

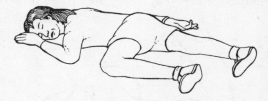

Warning: If you suspect that a casualty has a fractured spine or if they have fractures of the limbs, do not move them into the recovery position unless it becomes essential in order to preserve breathing.

CLEARING AND OPENING THE AIRWAY

The airway is the passage, from the nose and mouth to the lungs, by which air enters and leaves the lungs. If it is blocked, breathing will cease. Therefore it is essential to keep the airway clear and open.

Action

1 Place the casualty in the recovery position (see p. 8).
2 Gently check the mouth for vomit, foreign objects or broken teeth, and clear these away with your fingers. Remove dentures only if they are broken or loose.

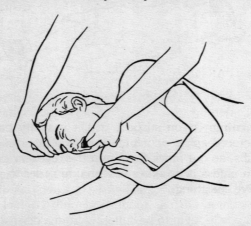

3 Keep the airway open so that breathing can occur, gently tilt the casualty's head back, with one of your

hands on the forehead and the point of the chin supported with the other.

CHECKING FOR BREATHING

Breathing should be regular, quiet and easy.

Action
1 **Look** for the rise and fall of the lower chest and abdomen. If there is no movement, the airway may be obstructed (see CHOKING).
2 **Listen and feel** for air escaping through the nose and mouth, by placing your face close to the casualty's.
3 If the casualty is not breathing, begin AR (see below) immediately.

GIVING ARTIFICIAL RESPIRATION (AR)

Mouth-to-mouth resuscitation is the easiest, most successful method of AR. Mouth-to-nose resuscitation is used when there is serious jaw injury or if the casualty has to be revived in deep water. Mouth-and-nose resuscitation is used for babies and small children when your mouth can cover both the mouth and the nose. Mouth-to-mask resuscitation used by a person trained in this technique avoids mouth-to-mouth contact if the casualty is thought to be suffering from a disease, such as hepatitis A or B or AIDS (acquired immunodeficiency syndrome), that can be transmitted to another person by blood or other body fluids; however, because the risk of catching such a disease is low for the person giving first aid, AR should not be withheld in the absence of a mask.

Action

Mouth-to-mouth Resuscitation

1 Kneel beside the casualty.
2 Place the casualty on his or her back.
3 Tilt the head back gently, supporting the jaw with your fingers. **Do not** press on the throat. The casualty's mouth should be only partly open.
4 Pinch the casualty's nostrils. Take a deep breath and place your mouth over the casualty's, sealing off any opening.

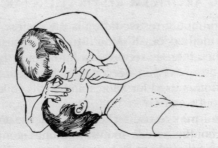

5 Keeping the casualty's head tilted, give 5 full breaths in 10 seconds.

6 Check the carotid pulse (see p. 16). If there is no pulse begin CPR (see p. 17).

7 If there is a pulse, check the casualty's breathing. Put your face close to his or her mouth and listen and feel for air being exhaled.

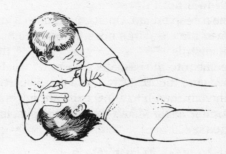

8 If there is no apparent breathing, continue AR, first checking that the head is tilted back far enough, the mouth and nose are sealed off so that no air escapes and the airway is clear. (If the stomach is distended, this may indicate a blocked airway.) Give 1 breath every 4 seconds.

9 After 1 minute check the pulse and breathing again and continue to do so every 2 minutes.

10 When the casualty is breathing again, place him or her in the recovery position (see p. 8) and check the airway, breathing and pulse frequently.

Mouth-to-nose Resuscitation

1 Kneel beside the casualty.
2 Place the casualty on his or her back, with the head tilted back.
3 Supporting the jaw with your fingers, close the casualty's mouth, and keep it closed, using your thumb on the lower lip.
4 Take a deep breath. Open your mouth wide and place it over the casualty's nose, without compressing the soft nostrils.
5 Breathe into the casualty's nose.
6 Move your mouth away. Open the casualty's lower lip with your thumb to allow exhalation.
7 Continue as for Mouth-to-mouth Resuscitation, steps 5–10 (see above).

Mouth-to-mask Resuscitation

1 Kneel either beside the casualty's head or at the top of the head facing the feet.
2 Place the narrow end of the mask on the bridge of the casualty's nose. Use both of your hands, placed on either side of the jaw, to keep the airway open and to hold the mask firmly in place, creating an airtight seal.

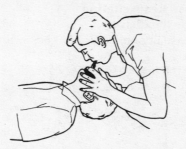

3 Take a deep breath and blow through the mouthpiece of the mask.

4 Remove your mouth to allow exhalation.

5 Continue as for Mouth-to-mouth Resuscitation, steps 5–10 (see pp. 12–13).

Mouth-and-nose Resuscitation (Babies and Children Under 8)

1 After clearing the airway, lay the child on his or her back, with the head horizontal, not tilted, and the jaw supported by your hand.

2 Place your mouth over the child's nose and slightly opened mouth. Puff gently, providing just enough air to make the child's chest rise.

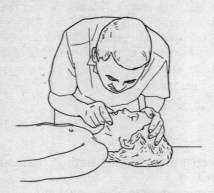

3 Continue as for Mouth-to-mouth Resuscitation, steps 5–10 (see pp. 12–13), but giving 1 shallow breath every 3 seconds.

CHECKING FOR PULSE

The pulse rate is the rate of the heart beat: 60–80 strong, regular beats per minute is normal for adults; up to 100 for a child; and up to 140 for a baby. When the heart stops beating, the blood in the body stops circulating. Breathing will stop and the casualty will be unconscious.

The carotid pulse should always be checked if the casualty is unconscious or seriously ill or injured.

Action
1 Lightly place the tips of your middle two or three

fingers on the casualty's Adam's apple, then slide them into the groove between it and the large neck muscle. **Feel only one side** when taking the pulse; it is easier to feel the pulse on the far side of the neck.

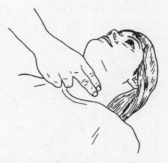

2 Feel for the pulse for 5 seconds.
3 If no pulse is present, begin CPR (see below) immediately.

CARDIOPULMONARY RESUSCITATION (CPR)

CPR is a combination of AR and external cardiac compression (ECC), or chest compression. It maintains an artificial circulation until expert help arrives.

CPR is very tiring and ideally should be carried out by two people to maintain the correct rhythm.

Action

CPR for Adults

1 Kneel beside the upper body and head of the casualty.
2 Leave the casualty on his or her back.
3 Locate the middle of the breastbone: find where the rib margins meet the bottom of the breastbone.

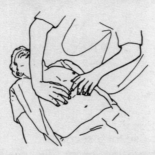

4 Position the heel of your hand at a width of two fingers above this point.
5 Place your hand that is nearer the casualty's head on top of your other hand, interlocking its fingers with those of the lower one or locking its thumb around the wrist of the lower one.

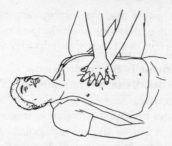

6 Keep your arms straight and, using the heel of your lower hand, depress the breastbone about 4–5cm, without exerting any pressure on the ribs. Release the pressure, allowing the chest to expand, but do not remove your hands. Continue the compressions, rhythmically depressing and releasing.

If you are alone: depress the breastbone 15 times in 10–12 seconds, then apply AR, giving 2 breaths in 3–5 seconds.

If you have help: one person should administer ECC, then allow the other person to give AR. Give 5 compressions, then 1 breath, in 5 seconds. The person applying compression needs to count the compressions out loud so that, at the end of the fifth one, AR is given by the other helper without any pause.

7 Check the pulse after 1 minute, then every 2 minutes. If there is no pulse, continue CPR. If there is a pulse but breathing has not returned, stop CPR and start AR.

8 When both pulse and breathing resume, place the casualty in the recovery position (see p. 8), and wait with the person until medical help arrives.

CPR for Children 1–8 Years

1 Find the middle of the breastbone (see CPR for Adults, steps 1–3, p. 18).

2 Place the heel of your hand that is nearer the child's abdomen just below the middle point of the breastbone, with your fingers relaxed, slightly raised and pointing across the chest.

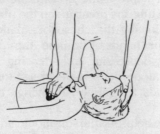

3 **Using only this heel**, and not the other hand as well, depress the chest about 2–3 cm, working gently and rhythmically.

If you are alone: give 15 compressions, then 2 quick shallow breaths, in 10 seconds.

If you have help: give 5 compressions, then 1 quick, shallow breath, in 3 seconds.

CPR for Babies

1 Find the middle of the breastbone (see CPR for Adults, steps 1–3, p. 18).
2 To apply compression **use only the index and middle fingers** of your hand on the lower half of the breastbone. Depress the chest lightly about 1.5 cm.

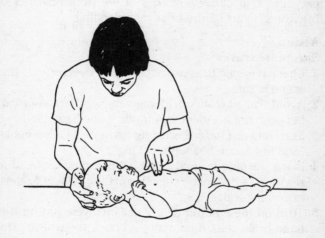

If you are alone: give 15 compressions, then 2 quick shallow breaths, in 10 seconds.

If you have help: give 5 compressions, then 1 quick, shallow breath, in 3 seconds.

ROAD TRAFFIC ACCIDENTS

Immediate, efficient first aid at a road accident is essential. The first few minutes are vital and prompt action can prevent brain damage or loss of life from obstructed breathing, heart failure or severe bleeding.

Action
Safety Measures
1 Check it is safe to approach and that everyone on the scene is safe.
2 Avoid danger from oncoming vehicles. Park your car between the accident and traffic if necessary.
3 Turn on your hazard warning lights or flashing lights (and low-beam headlights at night).
4 Place warning triangles and people, if possible, at a reasonable distance either side of the accident to alert oncoming traffic.
5 Turn off the ignition of any car involved, put on the hand brake and, if on a slope, chock the wheels. **Do not** touch a car or casualties if they are in contact with live electric cables; contact the electricity emergency service immediately. **Do not** right an overturned vehicle.
6 Check for flammable liquids, such as petrol, have fire extinguishers handy and **do not** smoke.

First Aid

1 Check if there are any casualties in the wreckage or by the side of the road. **Do not** smash a car window to get at a trapped casualty unless he or she is protected.

2 **Do not** move anyone unless he or she is in immediate danger. Try to give a trapped casualty first aid on the spot: slide or tilt the car seat back if the steering wheel or any other heavy object is compressing the chest; tilt the casualty's head back and support the jaw so that the airway remains open. If you must move someone, follow the instructions given in the next chapter, MOVING A CASUALTY.

3 Assess the condition of the casualties. **Remember**: treat an unconscious person first and immediately check the airway, breathing and circulation (see EMERGENCY PRIORITIES AND EMERGENCY TECHNIQUES), then stop any severe BLEEDING.

4 Send for help immediately. **Remember**: do not leave a seriously injured or unconscious casualty, unless help is unlikely to come, and always give clear, brief instructions about the location and nature of the accident (see EMERGENCY PRIORITIES).

MOVING A CASUALTY

Do not move an injured person unless there is immediate danger from fire, oncoming traffic or toxic fumes, for example. It is best to apply first aid on the spot and wait for medical help to arrive.

However, if you (and others) must move someone, remember to:

- hold the casualty firmly but gently
- take special care always to support the head, neck and spine, especially if the casualty is unconscious
- carry out the move smoothly, without jerking the casualty.

DRAGGING

This technique can be used in an emergency if the casualty is unconscious or seriously injured and you have no help.

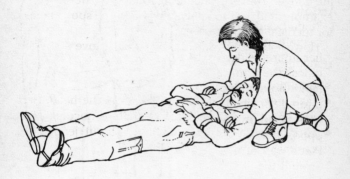

Action
1 Fold the casualty's arms across their chest.
2 Grasp the casualty underneath the armpits and drag.
3 While dragging, cradle their head on your arms.

HUMAN CRUTCH

This is suitable for an injured adult who can move with some help.

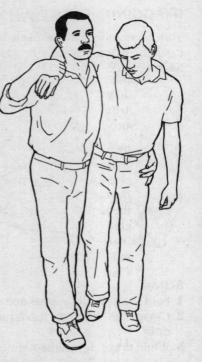

Action
1 Stand beside the casualty on his or her injured side, unless the arm, hand or shoulder is injured (in which case stand on the opposite side).
2 Place your arm around the casualty's back and grasp the clothing on the far hip.
3 Bring the casualty's arm around your neck, support him or her with your shoulder and hold the hand (unless it is seriously wounded or bleeding).
4 Move forward slowly with the casualty, both taking the first step with the inside foot.

FIRST AID KITS

A properly equipped first aid kit can save vital minutes in an emergency. In addition to your first aid kit at home, keep one in your car and boat and take a portable kit on camping trips and holidays.

Make sure you:

- label the kit 'First Aid'
- use a container that is childproof and waterproof
- replace items as they are used, do not keep medications for any length of time and safely dispose of a prescribed medicine once the course of treatment is completed
- tape a card, listing emergency phone numbers and the blood group, allergies and special medical problems of family members, to the container
- keep the kit handy but beyond the reach of children
- keep this book close by the kit for quick reference.

HOME KIT

A first aid kit for a family should contain the following:

- adhesive dressing strips for minor cuts and grazes
- adhesive tape to hold dressings in place

- analgesic tablets, such as paracetamol, for headaches and minor pain
- antihistamine cream for bites and stings
- antiseptic cream
- antiseptic solution
- cotton buds
- disposable gloves
- eye bath
- measuring glass or spoon
- plastic cup
- roller bandages in a range of sizes
- round-ended scissors (use only for first aid)
- safety pins
- splinter forceps or remover
- sterile combine dressing for severe bleeding
- sterile eye pads, wrapped singly
- sterile gauze swabs for cleaning wounds
- sterile non-adherent absorbent dressing for burns
- thermometer in a protective case
- triangular bandages
- tubular gauze finger bandage with applicator.

CAR KIT

Remember always to keep a copy of *Family First Aid* in your glove box. Your car kit should contain at least a selection of the dressings, pads and bandages listed above, scissors and safety pins.

DRESSINGS, PADS AND BANDAGES

DRESSINGS

A dressing is a protective cover placed over a wound, before it is bandaged, to help:

- control and absorb bleeding and discharge
- relieve pain
- prevent infection and further injury
- stop swelling.

A variety of sterile, non-adhesive dressings can be bought, but any clean, absorbent material that does not stick, such as cotton, linen, gauze or towelling, is suitable.

Do not apply cotton wool or fluffy material directly to a wound, because the fibres will stick.

Do not touch the wound or any part of the dressing that will be in contact with the wound.

PADS

Pads, made from layers of cloth, gauze or bandages, are sometimes placed over a dressing to apply pressure, increase the absorption of fluids or help protect skin.

Ring Pad

A ring pad holds a bandage away from a wound if there is an object embedded in the wound or a broken bone protruding through the skin.

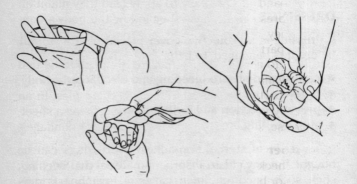

To make a ring pad: wind one end of a narrow bandage around your fingers to make a loop, then bring the other end through the loop and pass it over and under until a firm ring has been made.

BANDAGES

Bandages are used to:

- control bleeding
- keep dressings and pads in place
- help reduce or prevent swelling
- support a limb or joint, relieving pain

- restrict movement and, when used with SPLINTS, immobilise a limb or joint.

Ready-made bandages, usually of calico, crepe or gauze, are available. Modern crepe, elasticated or conforming bandages are easy to apply, and they maintain an even pressure because they follow the body's contours. They are available in a variety of widths for different parts of the body. Tubular gauze bandages are also easy to apply because they do not need to be tied and are available in sizes to fit different parts of the body; they are particularly useful for fingers and toes. In an emergency you can, however, improvise, using a sheet, pillow-case, stockings or other materials for bandages.

Remember

Always check that bandages are not too tight. Swelling, paleness or blueness of fingers or toes, numbness, 'pins and needles', pain and lack of a pulse in the part of the body below the bandage area are indications that bandages should be loosened. Bandaging must be checked regularly.

Triangular Bandages

These versatile calico or cotton bandages, with two sides approximately 90–100 cm long, can be used to cover a large dressing; as a pad; as SLINGS; to attach SPLINTS to limbs; and to protect the scalp, shoulder, hand, chest, foot or back. They can be folded into wide or narrow bandages.

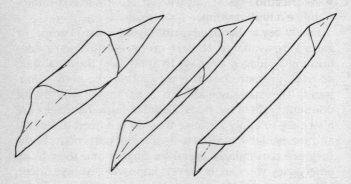

To make a narrow bandage from a triangular bandage: fold the point of the triangle over to meet the base edge, then fold the bandage over again. For a very narrow bandage, fold the bandage one more time.

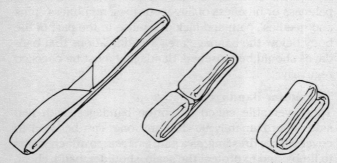

To make a pad from a folded triangular bandage: turn both ends in to meet at the middle, repeat the process and then fold one half of the layered bandage over the other.

Roller Bandages

Traditionally these have been made of linen, cotton or gauze. They are applied as follows:

1 Place yourself opposite the casualty.
2 Support the injured limb.
3 Hold the roll in one hand and bandage outwards from the casualty's body, working from below the injury to above it.

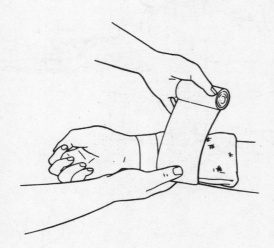

4 Overlap each turn by two-thirds and try to maintain even pressure. Finish with two or three turns above the wound.

5 Cut the roll, tuck the end of the bandage under and pin or tape. Alternatively, cut the end into two strips and tie them in a reef knot.

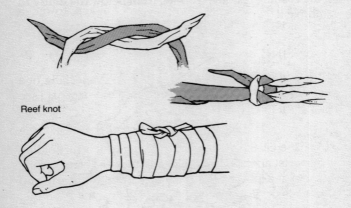

Reef knot

SLINGS

The purpose of a sling is to support, protect or immobilise an injured limb. Ready-made slings may be bought, but they can also be made from a triangular bandage (see DRESSINGS, PADS AND BANDAGES), a towel, a pillowcase, a scarf or other materials.

ARM SLING

An arm sling supports an injured arm (especially one with a SPLINT), such as a fractured forearm or wrist (see FRACTURES).

Action
1 Ask the casualty to support the injured arm, holding the wrist and hand a little higher than the elbow, while you place a triangular bandage between the arm and the chest, its point beyond the elbow.

2 Take the top end of the triangular bandage over the shoulder on the uninjured side and around the neck.

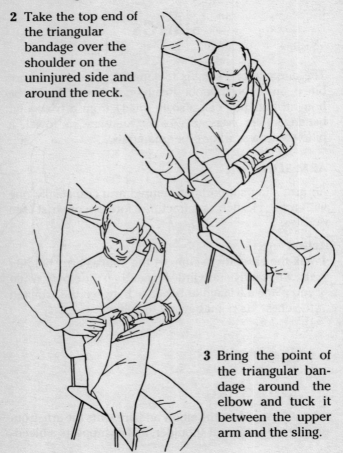

3 Bring the point of the triangular bandage around the elbow and tuck it between the upper arm and the sling.

4 Take the bottom end of the triangular bandage up over the hand and arm to meet the top end on the injured side. Tie the two ends in a reef knot (see DRESSINGS, PADS AND BANDAGES) in the hollow above the collar bone. Secure the sling at the elbow fold, with a safety pin.

5 Keep the casualty's nails free and check them regularly; if they are turning blue or white, loosen the sling a little.

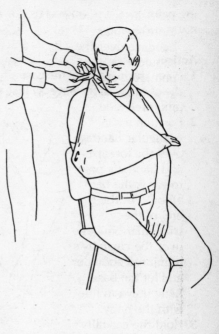

ELEVATION SLING

This sling supports the elbow and prevents the arm from pulling on an injured shoulder. It also supports a bleeding palm (see CUTS AND WOUNDS), or a fractured hand (see FRACTURES).

Action

1 Place the forearm of the casualty's injured arm across the chest, with the fingers close to the shoulder on the uninjured side.
2 Position a triangular bandage over the forearm and hand, its point towards the bent elbow. Put the top end of the triangular bandage over the casualty's uninjured shoulder and let the base hang down in line with the body.
3 Hold the casualty's hand and the top end of the triangular bandage over the uninjured shoulder and tuck the triangular bandage under the casualty's hand and wrist, with your thumb.

4 With your other hand, tuck the point of the triangular bandage firmly under the casualty's upper arm. Next, sweep the same hand under the part of the triangular bandage still hanging down, and bring it up under the upper arm, tucking in the folds.

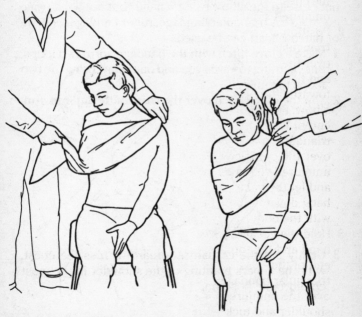

5 Bring the end across the casualty's back and tie it and the other end in a reef knot in the hollow above the collar bone on the uninjured side. Secure the elbow fold, with a safety pin.

COLLAR-AND-CUFF SLING

This is a suitable sling either for an upper arm fracture not close to the elbow or for a hand (but not wrist) (see FRACTURES). A triangular bandage, roller bandage, belt, tie or narrow scarf can be used.

1 Make a clove hitch with the bandage: form two loops, one pointing towards you and one away; bring the two loops together.
2 Slip the clove hitch over the wrist of the injured arm.

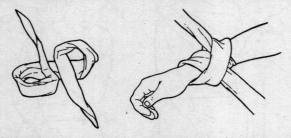

3 Gently put the casualty's forearm across the chest, with the fingers pointing to the shoulder in the most comfortable position.

4 Take the ends of the sling around the neck and tie them in a reef knot in the hollow above either collar bone.

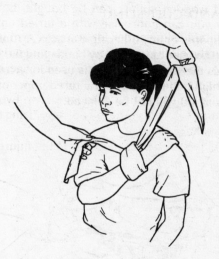

SPLINTS

Splints are used to protect wounds from further injury and to support or immobilise limbs in cases of a fractured upper or lower leg if medical aid will be delayed.

They should also be used for a fractured kneecap, upper arm close to the elbow, forearm, wrist or finger (see FRACTURES).

Prepared wooden splints can be bought, but in an emergency you can improvise with a furled umbrella, rolled newspaper or any other rigid article. An uninjured leg can also be used as a splint by bandaging the injured leg to it; this method of splinting is used for a fractured neck of a thigh bone, and for a fractured upper or lower leg if medical aid will not be delayed.

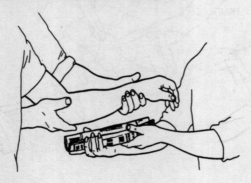

Remember
- Move the injured limb as little as possible while applying the splint.
- The splint should be rigid and long enough to extend beyond the joints on either side of the fracture.

- Check bandages every 15 minutes to ensure blood circulation is not being restricted.

Action

1 Pad the splint well, using clean material, folded bandages or whatever is at hand. Use extra padding between the splint and the natural hollows and bony areas, such as ankles and wrists.

2 Firmly tie the splint to the limb at the top and the bottom, using bandages. **Do not** bandage directly over FRACTURES.

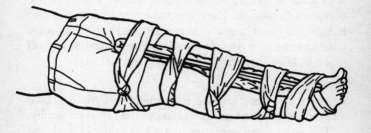

FAMILY SAFETY

The home is a dangerous place to be. Every year many children die from accidents at home. Thousands more people, of all ages, are scarred or disabled for life. Elderly people as well as children are particularly prone to accidents.

The kitchen is the home's most dangerous room. It is the place where family members usually spend the most time and where most accidents occur. Children are particularly at risk. They are naturally inquisitive and inclined to touch and try everything and to hang around your knees when you are cooking. The kitchen is a good place to keep your first aid kit (see FIRST AID KITS).

Remember

- There are many simple, easy measures you can take that will prevent accidents happening to your family. The following checklists will allow you to check the safety of your home and children and give you ideas for improving family safety.

KITCHEN CHECKLIST

- Keep all appliances and power points well out of children's reach. Insert dummy plugs in low power points.

- Do not allow the cords of electric appliances to trail, especially (not) near the sink or stove.
- Always unplug the electric kettle before filling it with water.
- Keep full teapots and hot drinks well away from the edge of tables and benches, and never pass a hot drink over a child's head.
- Store knives safely.
- Switch the iron off as soon as you have finished and leave it in a safe place to cool down.
- Keep matches and lighters out of the reach of small children, and teach older children about their dangers and how to use them safely.
- Do not allow the tablecloth to hang over the edge of the table when a baby or toddler is present.
- Keep all cleaning products out of the reach of children, particularly dishwasher detergent, oven cleaner, bleach and corrosive chemicals. **Do not** store them under the kitchen sink unless the cupboard is kept locked at all times.
- Store plastic bags well out of reach of children: suffocation can take place quickly and silently.

COOKING CHECKLIST

- Take special care when cooking with oil, which can spatter and burn a bystander or catch fire (nearly half of all house fires start in the kitchen). **If a pan**

catches on fire, cover it with a lid or damp cloth. Leave it where it is until it cools down.

- Never pour water into hot oil: the burst of steam resulting can easily scald.
- Wipe up food spilt on the floor immediately to avoid the family slipping on it.
- Place pots and pans on the back burners whenever possible and keep all handles turned inwards. A stove safety guard is a good investment if you have children.
- Encourage children to stay well clear of the stove when you are cooking. Take a few minutes, before you start, to give them something to do in a safe area: for example, reading, games or drawing.

BATHROOM CHECKLIST

- Have wiring in the bathroom professionally fitted: water and electricity are a dangerous combination.
- Always double check the water temperature before putting a baby or child in the bath. Always put the cold water in first.
- Take special care if you use an electric shaver or hair dryer in the bathroom. It is better to use a hair dryer in the bedroom, well away from water.
- Do not use a portable heater in the bathroom. Have a safe heater professionally installed.
- Never leave a baby or child alone in the bath. **If you**

must answer the phone or door, wrap the child in a towel and take him or her with you.

- Use non-skid mats in the bath and shower, and install safety rails for children or elderly people to hold on to.
- Keep medicines, the first aid kit, cosmetics and perfumes out of the reach of children.
- Keep scissors, razor blades and electric shavers out of the reach of children.
- Teach everyone in the family not to touch power points with wet hands; moisture is an excellent conductor of electricity.
- Keep lavatory cleaners, bleach and other cleaners out of the reach of children.

GARDEN CHECKLIST

- Always wear gloves when you are gardening. They prevent cuts from glass and rusty metal or nails.
- Use poisonous weed-killers and sprays as little as possible. There are efficient non-toxic and herbal products available.
- Correctly label all fertilisers, weed-killers and poisons and keep out of the reach of children.
- Wear shoes (ideally sturdy ones) when you are mowing or using an electric garden appliance, such as clippers.

- Keep rubbish bins well sealed so that children cannot rummage through them.
- Never leave a child unattended near a swimming pool. Always empty paddling pools after use and store them away. **Remember**: a child can drown in just a few inches of water.

CHILD SAFETY CHECKLIST

Note that drowning and choking are common causes of accidental death in young children. Burns are also a common accident.

- Never give peanuts to a child under 3.
- Never leave a baby alone with food or drink: it can choke and die in minutes.
- Do not tie a dummy with a ribbon or string around the baby's neck as it can become entangled and cause strangulation.
- Do not leave plastic bags lying around. Put them away immediately and teach children that they are not toys to play with.
- Ensure that all baby equipment is safe and conforms to approved safety standards. Take special care when purchasing cots, high-chairs, play-pens, prams and strollers.
- Always supervise a child in a high-chair.
- Place a safety guard around a fire or radiator.
- Always use a child's car seat that is approved by the

standards association and make sure that it is **fitted correctly**, and **adjust safety belts and harnesses** every time you take a baby or child in your car.

- Never keep a baby in a car on a hot day.
- Never leave a baby or child unattended in a car.
- Teach your child about road safety. Every time you cross the road, hold your child's hand and explain the correct procedure. Whenever possible, cross at a pedestrian crossing or traffic lights.

A TO Z OF INJURIES
AND ILLNESSES

ASTHMA ATTACK

Asthma is one of the most common chronic childhood diseases in the UK. It affects around 5% of the total population and about 10% of children. Any child who experiences persistent shortness of breath, wheeziness or cough may be a potential asthmatic and should see a doctor.

During an attack, the muscle surrounding the air tubes goes into spasm, the lining of the tubes becomes swollen and excessive mucus is produced, all of which results in the tubes narrowing, making breathing difficult.

Most asthma sufferers carry their own medication, usually in the form of a metered-dose, bronchodilator aerosol, such as Ventolin, commonly known as a 'puffer'. Children under 5 may need to use other devices.

Signs and Symptoms
- difficulty breathing
- rapid, shallow breaths
- noisy, wheezy breathing
- coughing
- feeling of tightness in the chest
- difficulty speaking, moving and eating, in severe attacks
- blueness of lips and confusion, in very severe cases
- in severe attacks breathing may sound quiet.

Warning

The seriousness of an asthma attack is difficult to assess and varies, but occasionally asthma is fatal, so prompt action should always be taken.

If the sufferer is not carrying medication, medical aid should be sought immediately: the quickest way to do this is to call an ambulance because all ambulances are equipped to deal with asthma in young children and others.

Action

1 Sit the sufferer in a quiet, warm place, away from other people and leaning on a table.

2 Give the sufferer 4–6 puffs from his or her puffer, one after another.

3 Wait 10 minutes and then, if there is no improvement, give 4–6 more puffs.

4 If there is still no improvement, call an ambulance immediately.

5 While waiting for medical help to arrive, continue to administer the puffer as given in steps 2–3. Note that these bronchodilator puffers are safe to use and that an overdose is very unlikely. Oxygen should also be given at this stage if it is available.

BITES AND STINGS

Bites and stings can cause great discomfort and can sometimes also need medical attention. Stitches, antibiotics or a tetanus injection may be required after an animal bite. Some people suffer an allergic reaction to what would normally be just a painful bite or sting, in some cases the reaction is severe and must be treated immediately (see Bees and Wasps, below).

BITES

Action
1 Wash the wound thoroughly with a mild antiseptic or soap and water.
2 Cover the wound with a clean dressing and bandage (see DRESSINGS, PADS AND BANDAGES).
3 Seek medical aid, unless the wound is superficial, because antibiotics or stitches may be required. The sufferer may also require a tetanus injection unless one has recently been administered.

BEES AND WASPS

Some people suffer allergic reactions to the sting of bees and wasps.

Signs and Symptoms of Allergic Reaction
- local pain, swelling and itchiness
- itchy rash on the body
- puffy eyelids and face
- constricted throat and difficulty breathing

Action
1 If a bee sting is involved, remove the sting by brushing it sideways with your fingernail or a knife blade. **Do not** squeeze the poison sac by pulling out the barb.
2 Wipe the area and apply a cold compress.
3 If there is an allergic reaction, the casualty should immediately take any medication for allergy that he or she may be carrying. If the reaction is severe, monitor breathing, begin AR if necessary (see EMERGENCY TECHNIQUES) and seek medical aid urgently.

BLEEDING

Severe or continued bleeding, if not controlled, is potentially fatal. It is critical to stop the bleeding as quickly as possible.

Internal bleeding can occur after a serious accident or heavy fall or result from a medical condition, such as a stomach ulcer. Bleeding into the tissues and cavities of the body can be life-threatening, and immediate hospital care is essential.

EXTERNAL BLEEDING

Signs and Symptoms
- bleeding from a wound
- SHOCK

Action
1 Lay the casualty down (unless there are CHEST INJURIES).
2 Check that the wound does not contain a foreign body or protruding bone (see FRACTURES). If it does, **do not** disturb it, but apply a ring pad (see DRESSINGS, PADS AND BANDAGES).

3 If the wound is clear of protruding matter, apply direct pressure immediately to it: use your hands until you can add a clean dressing and pad.

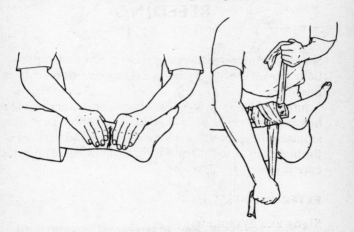

4 Bandage the wound firmly. If it is on an arm or leg and there are no obvious fractures, raise the limb.

5 If blood seeps through the bandage, leave the dressing in place but replace the pad. **Do not** remove the dressing, pad or bandage when bleeding stops.

6 **Do not** give anything to eat or drink.

7 Monitor the casualty for shock.

8 Seek medical aid urgently.

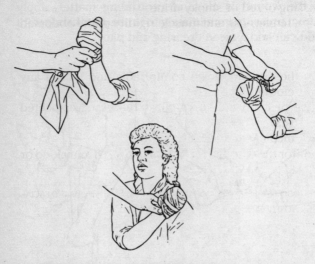

To stop bleeding from the palm, which can be severe: get the casualty to grip a pad in the palm to apply pressure to the wound; elevate the hand; leaving one end at the base of the thumb, take a bandage around the hand, down over the fist and around and over the thumb and end of bandage, continue bandaging in this way, then tie both ends at the top of the fist; finally, rest the bandaged hand against the shoulder on the uninjured side and support it with an elevation sling (see SLINGS).

INTERNAL BLEEDING

Signs and Symptoms

- coughing or vomiting up of blood
- passing of black or red faeces

- passing of red or smoky urine
- pain, tenderness and muscle rigidity of the abdomen
- SHOCK

Action

1 Lay the casualty down comfortably and loosen any tight clothing.
2 Raise or bend the legs (unless there are suspected FRACTURES).
3 Seek medical aid urgently.
4 Monitor the casualty for SHOCK. **Do not** give any food or drink.

See also BRUISES; CUTS AND WOUNDS; EAR INJURIES; HEAD AND FACIAL INJURIES; NOSEBLEED.

BRUISES

A heavy fall or blow can cause bleeding beneath the skin.

Signs and Symptoms

- pain
- bruise, which turns from red to bluish purple to greenish yellow
- swelling
- tenderness

Action

1 Check for injuries, particularly FRACTURES, SPRAINS AND DISLOCATIONS OR STRAINS.
2 Apply an ice pack (see SPRAINS AND DISLOCATIONS).
3 Rest the casualty, support the injured part and apply a compression bandage. A heavily bruised arm should be supported with a sling (see SLINGS). If the legs or body are bruised, support them with cushions.

For the treatment of a black eye see EYE INJURIES.

BURNS AND SCALDS

Burns are caused by the dry heat from flames, electricity, lightning, chemicals and radiation (for example, in sunburn). Scalds are caused by moist heat from boiling liquids or steam. Burns and scalds are serious injuries and can result in infection, scarring and, in extreme cases, death.

Signs and Symptoms

- skin looks red and blistered if only the outer layers are affected
- skin looks dark red, blackened or charred if all the layers of skin are burnt
- pain if the burn or scald is superficial, but it may be absent if nerve ends have been damaged
- SHOCK if burns or scalds are extensive

Action

1 Remove the casualty from danger and the source of heat if you can do so without becoming a casualty yourself (see MOVING A CASUALTY).

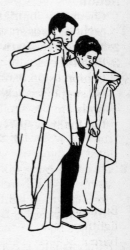

2 If the casualty's clothes are on fire, protect yourself by holding a blanket or rug in front of yourself as you approach him or her. Wrap the blanket or rug around the casualty to smother the flames, and lay him or her on the ground. If you must use water to put out the flames, **do not** throw it.

3 If the casualty is unconscious, place him or her in the recovery position, check the airway, breathing

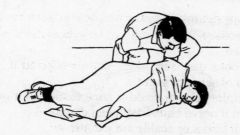

and pulse and begin AR or CPR if necessary (see EMERGENCY TECHNIQUES).

4 Carefully remove clothing, jewellery, etc. from the affected area; **do not** remove any item that is stuck to the burn.

5 Cool the burnt area with cold, but not icy, water, ideally by placing the burn under gently running water for at least 10 minutes.

6 Cover the burn with a sterile, non-adherent dressing, then lightly apply a bandage (see DRESSINGS, PADS AND BANDAGES). **Do not** apply ointments, lotions or cream.

7 If the casualty is conscious and thirsty, give him or her water to sip slowly. **Do not** give alcohol.

8 Rest the casualty comfortably, supporting any burnt limb.

9 For all except minor burns and scalds, seek medical aid immediately.

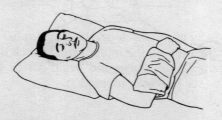

CHEST INJURIES

The chest protects the heart, lungs and major blood vessels, so injuries to this area can quickly affect breathing and circulation and may result in profuse BLEEDING.

Sometimes a fractured rib may pierce the lung, causing serious damage, internal bleeding or even the collapse of the lung.

If a fractured rib or a sharp object has penetrated the chest wall, air from outside can be sucked directly into the chest cavity. This air can cause the lung on the injured side to collapse.

FRACTURED RIBS

Signs and Symptoms
- pain, worsening when the casualty breathes or coughs
- difficulty breathing
- frothy blood coughed up, sometimes
- tenderness in the injury area

Action
1 If the casualty is unconscious, place him or her in the recovery position on the injured side, check the airway, breathing and pulse and begin AR or CPR if necessary (see EMERGENCY TECHNIQUES).

2 Rest the conscious casualty in a half-sitting position, leaning downwards on the injured side.

3 Pad the injured side, then bandage the upper arm and padding to the injured side (see DRESSINGS, PADS AND BANDAGES).

4 Immobilise the arm with an elevation or collar-and-cuff sling (see SLINGS).

5 Seek medical aid urgently.

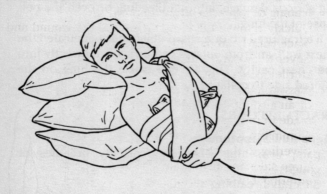

SUCKING WOUNDS

Signs and Symptoms
- pain in the area of the injury
- blood bubbling from the wound
- bluish lips
- increasing difficulty breathing

- sucking noise from the wound
- unconsciousness

Action

1 If casualty is unconscious, place him or her in the recovery position on the injured side, check the airway, breathing and pulse and begin AR or CPR if necessary (see EMERGENCY TECHNIQUES).

2 Rest the conscious casualty in a half-sitting position, leaning downwards on the injured side.

3 Quickly remove the clothing around the wound and place your hand over the wound.

4 Cover the wound with a sterile dressing (see DRESSINGS, PADS AND BANDAGES) or an airtight dressing made from plastic or aluminium foil. Tape the covering to the chest on three sides to prevent air entering, but **do not** tape the bottom edge – leave it open so that air under pressure can escape.

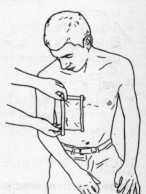

5 Seek medical aid urgently.

CHOKING

A piece of food, fishbone or other object can lodge in the airway, obstructing breathing. Young children can choke on a peanut or a part of a toy. Choking is potentially fatal and immediate first aid is essential.

PARTIALLY BLOCKED AIRWAY

Signs and Symptoms
- coughing
- difficulty breathing
- blueness of the face, neck and extremities
- unconsciousness, sometimes

Warning
- If an adult, child or baby can cough, cry or walk do not slap him or her on the back because this can cause the obstruction to shift and become a total blockage of the airway.

Action
1 Place the unconscious, breathing casualty in the recovery position, monitoring the airway, breathing and pulse (see EMERGENCY TECHNIQUES) and seek medical aid urgently.
2 Encourage the conscious casualty to relax and allow

him or her to cough. If laboured breathing continues seek medical aid urgently.

COMPLETELY BLOCKED AIRWAY

Signs and Symptoms
- inability to cough
- inability to breathe
- unconsciousness
- the airway resists air and the chest fails to rise when AR is begun

Action
1 Position the casualty so that the head is slightly lower than the chest. Support a baby's chest and body across your knees. Place a child head down across your knee, with the chest supported by one hand.
2 Give 3–4 sharp slaps between the shoulder blades with your hand.
3 If this fails, attempt the Heimlich manoeuvre by standing or kneeling behind the person and

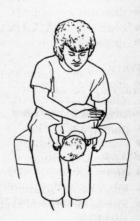

putting one arm around their abdomen with your fist just below the bottom of their breast bone. Place your other fist on top of the first fist and thrust hard upwards and inwards. Repeat if necessary.

Warning: This technique can be used on children, but use one fist or a couple of fingers only as there is a risk of damage to internal organs.

4 If there is no improvement, give AR (see EMERGENCY TECHNIQUES).

5 Seek medical aid urgently.

CONCUSSION

A severe fall or blow to the head or face can shake the brain and cause concussion.

Signs and Symptoms
- pale, clammy skin
- shallow breathing
- nausea, vomiting
- dizziness
- loss of consciousness, sometimes only momentary
- loss of memory of events shortly before or during the accident
- double vision

- headache
- SHOCK

Action

1 Lay the casualty down in a comfortable position. **Do not** give any food or drink.
2 Apply a cold compress to the knocked area.
3 Watch for any worsening of the condition.
4 If the casualty loses consciousness, place him or her in the recovery position, check the airway, breathing and pulse and begin AR or CPR if necessary (see EMERGENCY TECHNIQUES).
5 Seek medical advice: anyone who has lost consciousness because of a blow, even if only briefly, should see a doctor.

See also HEAD INJURIES.

CONVULSIONS

A convulsion is an episode in which normal brain activity becomes disturbed. It can be caused by a serious accident, DRUG OVERDOSE, fever or epilepsy.

Babies and young children, between the ages of 6 months and 6 years, can suffer seizures known as febrile convulsions. Febrile convulsions are caused by a sudden rise in body temperature associated with an infection that may or may not be obvious. Without complications, they do not cause damage or result in epilepsy.

Epilepsy is a disorder that takes the form of recurring seizures. The seizures occur as a result of a brief disturbance of electrochemical activity in the brain. There are many types of seizures. Major generalised (tonic-clonic or 'grand mal') seizure is one common type of epileptic seizure. Usually epileptic seizures are brief – lasting only a few seconds or minutes – and stop of their own accord. Most involve a change in consciousness. However, some seizures, such as the 'petit mal' (absence) seizure, which is a brief staring episode, are subtle and may go undiagnosed for years.

FEBRILE CONVULSIONS

Signs and Symptoms

The convulsion usually lasts only a few minutes and may involve:

- jerking or twitching of the body
- limpness of the body
- difficulty breathing
- unconsciousness

Action

1 Protect the child from injury by removing any dangerous objects, but **do not** forcibly restrain him or her.

2 During the seizure, place the child in the recovery position and keep the airway clear (see EMERGENCY TECHNIQUES).

3 Remove all the child's clothing and sponge him or her with tepid water to reduce the fever.

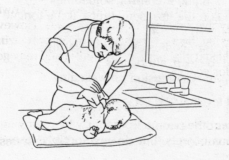

4 Fan the child to further assist the cooling process, but **do not** overcool.

5 Give the child a medicine, such as Calpol, to reduce the fever, following the instructions on the container.

6 Cover the child lightly once the TEMPERATURE has been reduced.

7 Seek medical aid before the temperature rises again.

EPILEPSY

Signs and Symptoms of Major Generalised Seizure

- person suddenly falls, rigid and unconscious, to the ground
- body convulses or shakes
- altered breathing pattern
- frothing at the mouth, sometimes
- loss of bladder control, sometimes
- blood on the lips, sometimes, if the tongue has been bitten
- temporary confusion on recovering
- need to sleep, afterwards
- temporary confusion on wakening

Action

1 Protect the person from injury by removing any dangerous objects, but **do not** forcibly restrain him or her.

2 As soon as the convulsions allow you, place the person in the recovery position and keep the airway clear (SEE EMERGENCY TECHNIQUE), but **do not** force anything into the mouth.

3 Place something soft under the person's head and loosen any tight clothing.

4 On recovery, help the person to somewhere nearby where he or she can rest or sleep. Allow the person to

recover naturally after full consciousness has returned.

5 Seek medical aid if the seizure lasts longer than 5 minutes in a child or 10 minutes in an adult, or if there are further seizures.

CRAMP

Cramp is a sudden and prolonged muscle contraction causing sharp pain. It may be caused by lack of body fluid (for example, after heavy vomiting or diarrhoea) or strenuous exercise in extremely hot or cold conditions.

Action

1 Gently stretch and straighten the cramped muscle: for hand cramp, get the sufferer to straighten the fingers and press down on the tips; for foot or calf cramp, have the sufferer stand, pushing down on the heel and toes; for thigh cramp, seat the person, straighten the leg, lift the toes with one of your hands and press down on the knee with your other one.

2 If cramp is due to loss of fluid, administer tepid water to which glucose or sugar has been added.

CUTS AND WOUNDS

Minor cuts, scratches and abrasions do not usually require medical attention. Abrasions, such as gravel rash, may have dirt embedded in the wound and are likely to become infected.

A stab or penetrating wound is caused by a sharp object, such as a knife, bullet, scissors blade or nail. Although the surface cut may be small, such objects can penetrate deeply and harm internal organs. These objects may also carry dirt deep inside, increasing the risk of infection.

CUTS AND ABRASIONS

Action

1 Wash your hands thoroughly before treating the wound.
2 Gently brush away any surface foreign object, such as gravel.
3 Clean the wound and surrounding area, wiping away from the wound, using sterile swabs, warm, sterile water and a little mild antiseptic. Pat the skin around the wound dry but do not wipe away blood clots.
4 Apply a sterile, non-adherent dressing if necessary (see DRESSINGS, PADS AND BANDAGES).
5 If the wound is dirty or caused by a rusty object, a tetanus injection may be needed.

STAB WOUNDS

Action

1 Stop any BLEEDING by applying direct pressure.
2 Cut away or remove the clothing around the wound.
3 Carefully cleanse the wound if it is not bleeding and apply a sterile dressing (see DRESSINGS, PADS AND BANDAGES).
4 If a limb is affected raise it, unless you suspect a fracture.
5 Seek medical aid.

WOUND WITH EMBEDDED OBJECT

Action

1 **Do not** attempt to remove the object. Apply a ring pad (see DRESSINGS, PADS AND BANDAGES) or pad around the wound and apply a clean dressing.
2 Apply pressure around the object to stop BLEEDING, but **do not** apply pressure to the object.
3 If a limb is affected raise it, unless you suspect a fracture.
4 Seek medical aid urgently.

SEVERED LIMBS

It may be possible to save a severed limb, finger or toe if you act quickly. Your first priority, however, is to save the casualty's life.

Warning
- Do not attempt to bandage a severed limb in position. You will cause further distress and pain to the casualty and damage delicate tissues, hampering possible micro-surgery.

Action
1 Lay the casualty down, with the injured part of the body supported in a raised position.
2 Firmly press a large piece of gauze or clean cloth against the stump or raw area to stop BLEEDING. Bandage the dressing in place.
3 Seek urgent medical aid.
4 Encourage the casualty to stay as still as possible. Watch closely for any signs of SHOCK, which can be caused by the loss of blood.
5 Find the severed limb and wrap it in clean gauze or cloth. **Do not** wash it. Place it in a watertight container, such as an inflated and sealed plastic bag. Put the container in water to which, if possible, ice has been added, but **do not** allow the part to have direct contact with the ice. Send the container to hospital with the casualty.

See also CHEST INJURIES; FISH HOOK INJURY; HEAD AND FACIAL INJURIES.

DIABETES

A person with diabetes has no insulin or insufficient amounts of insulin, produced by the pancreas, to maintain a balanced blood sugar level. Diabetes can be treated by a special diet, by a special diet and oral hypoglycaemic agents (tablets) or by a special diet and insulin therapy.

If a person with diabetes receives too much insulin or insufficient food while taking insulin, he or she can suffer from low blood sugar (hypoglycaemia) and become unconscious. If too little insulin is obtained, a high blood sugar level (hyperglycaemia) can cause a diabetic coma. However, a medical emergency is more likely to involve low blood sugar because high blood sugar usually develops over a greater length of time, so the person has more warning.

LOW BLOOD SUGAR

Signs and Symptoms
- faintness, giddiness of rapid onset
- hunger
- pale, sweating skin
- tingling around the mouth
- rapid pulse

- slurred speech
- mental confusion and perhaps aggressive behaviour
- weakness
- unconsciousness

Action

1 If the person is unconscious **do not** give anything by mouth; place him or her in the recovery position and check the airway, breathing and pulse (see EMERGENCY TECHNIQUES).
2 Seek medical help immediately.
3 If the person is conscious, give him or her glucose in the form of, for example, lemonade, orange juice, sweet tea or a glass of water with 2 teaspoons of sugar in it.
4 Once the person feels better (usually a few minutes after having the glucose), give him or her some complex carbohydrates, such as fruit or a sandwich.
5 Make sure the person discusses the possible causes of the hypoglycaemic episode with his or her doctor so that it may be avoided in the future.

HIGH BLOOD SUGAR

Signs and Symptoms

- extreme thirst
- need to urinate frequently
- tiredness, sleepiness
- dry, flushed skin

- rapid pulse
- deep breathing
- blurred vision
- nausea, vomiting, abdominal pain
- breath has a sweetish, acetone odour
- unconsciousness

Action

1 If the person is unconscious, place him or her in the recovery position, check the airway, breathing and pulse and begin AR or CPR if necessary (see EMERGENCY TECHNIQUES).

2 Seek medical aid urgently.

DROWNING

As a person struggles to stay afloat water can enter the airway, blocking the air supply. If breathing stops and the oxygen supply to the brain is cut off, permanent brain damage or death can result.

It is therefore vital to start AR as quickly as possible – as the person is being taken from the water if it is safe to do so.

Prevent drowning by:

- learning to swim

- teaching your children to swim
- not leaving children alone at a swimming pool or beach
- learning basic rescue and resuscitation procedures

Warning

- Do not attempt to rescue anyone in deep water if you are an inexperienced swimmer. Instead, call for help immediately.

Action

1 Check the airway, clearing it of vomit or any other obstruction, and begin mouth-to-nose AR (see EMERGENCY TECHNIQUES) while coming ashore in shallow water if it is safe to do so.

Do not
attempt
resuscitation
in deep water
unless you
have been
trained to do
so or are a
very strong
swimmer.

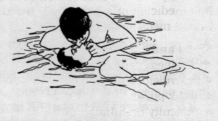

2 When the casualty is on firm ground, place him or her in the recovery position and check the airway again.

3 Start or resume AR.

4 When the casualty starts breathing again, maintain him or her in the recovery position, covered with a towel or blanket.

5 Seek medical aid immediately. Any person who has lost consciousness or been resuscitated must go to hospital.

6 Monitor the casualty's breathing and pulse closely until medical help arrives because relapses often occur.

DRUG OVERDOSE

This may involve an accidental overdose of a prescription medicine or a potentially lethal dose of narcotics. Urgent medical aid is needed.

Signs and Symptoms
- dizziness, faintness
- convulsions
- weak pulse
- difficulty breathing
- vomiting
- loss of consciousness

Note that signs and symptoms vary depending on the type and quantity of drug taken.

Action

1 If the casualty is unconscious, place him or her in the recovery position, check the airway, breathing and pulse and begin AR or CPR if necessary (see EMERGENCY TECHNIQUES). If breathing and pulse are satisfactory, maintain the unconscious person in the recovery position and continue to monitor breathing and pulse.

2 If the casualty is conscious, treat as for POISONING, but **do not** induce vomiting unless instructed to do so by your Poisons Information Centre or a doctor.

3 Try to establish which drug was taken, and send any containers, tablets or syringes to the hospital with the casualty. Also send a sample of vomit, in a covered jar.

4 Seek medical aid urgently.

EAR INJURIES

BLEEDING

Bleeding from the ear can indicate a serious head injury, such as a fractured skull, which can be life-threatening.

Action

1 Place the person in the recovery position (see EMER-GENCY TECHNIQUES), with the injured ear tilted down-

wards on a clean dressing to help the fluid drain. **Do
not** plug the ear or give drops.
2 Seek medical help urgently.

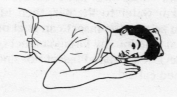

PERFORATED EARDRUM

The eardrum is a membrane, across the passage between the middle and outer ear, essential to hearing. A
ruptured eardrum can be caused by pressure changes, a
blow, explosions, a foreign agent or an infection.

Signs and Symptoms
● severe pain
● loss of hearing
● blood or fluid flow

Action
As for Bleeding (see above).

FOREIGN OBJECT

Small objects, such as beads or insects, can enter the
ear.

Action

1 **Do not** probe the ear. **Do not** attempt to remove any object unless it is an insect. If the object is an insect, tilt the person's head away from you and administer a drop of warm water to the ear, then tilt the head towards you so that the insect can float out.

2 Seek medical help for any foreign object other than a trapped insect. If a trapped insect does not float out, also seek medical aid.

ELECTRIC SHOCK

An electric shock can cause a mild 'pins and needles' sensation or can stop breathing and cause heart failure, resulting in death.

Frayed or faulty wires, defective appliances and appliances used near water are common but preventable causes of electric shock in the home.

Warning

• Before touching the victim make sure you are safe. Immediately turn off the current at the mains or power point and, if the accident involves an appliance, pull out the plug.

  In the case of high-voltage electricity, involving, for

example, electric train lines or heavy machinery, stay well clear, call for emergency help urgently and wait for trained personnel to disconnect the power.

Action

1 If you cannot turn off the power, move the casualty away from the source of electricity, using something dry and non-conducting, such as a wooden broom handle, a wooden chair or a rolled newspaper. Stand on a non-conducting surface (for example, a dry rubber mat or a newspaper) while you do this.

2 When the casualty is clear, smother the flames of any burning clothing (see BURNS AND SCALDS).

3 If the casualty is unconscious, place him or her in the recovery position, check the airway, breathing and pulse and begin AR or CPR if necessary (see EMERGENCY TECHNIQUES).

4 Treat any burns (see BURNS AND SCALDS).

5 Seek medical aid.

EYE INJURIES

The eye is extremely sensitive, delicate and susceptible to infection, so all injuries are potentially serious. Medical help should be sought as soon as possible to prevent permanent damage.

CHEMICAL AND HEAT BURNS

First aid treatment is needed immediately for burns from
chemicals, such as acids and caustic soda.

Signs and Symptoms
- pain
- sensitivity to light
- severe weeping of the eye
- reddened eyeballs
- swelling eyelids

Action
1 Open the casualty's eyelids gently with your fingers.
2 Flush the eye with gently running, cool water for at
   least 20 minutes.

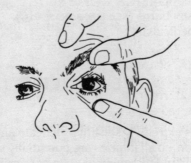

3 Apply a light, sterile dressing or eye pad to the eye.
4 Seek medical aid immediately.

FLASH BURNS

These can be caused by the flash from an arc welder.

Signs and Symptoms
- as for Chemical and Heat Burns (see above)
- a sensation of grit under the eyelids, which may be delayed

Action
1 **Do not** flush with water, instead apply a clean dressing or eye pad.
2 Seek medical aid.

SURFACE FOREIGN BODIES

An eyelash or speck of dust or other small particle can cause considerable discomfort.

Signs and Symptoms
- gritty feeling
- pain and irritation
- watery, red eye
- partially or completely closed eye
- sensitivity to light
- twitching eyelid

Warning

Do not attempt to remove a surface object from any part of the eye other than the white or eyelids.

- Do not attempt to remove the object if it is embedded in the eye (see below).

Action

1 Stop the sufferer from rubbing the eye.
2 Ask the person to look up. Gently hold the eyelids apart and try to remove the object, if visible, with the corner of a clean, moistened cloth.
3 If the object is not visible, have the sufferer look down. Gently take hold of the lashes of the upper lid and pull the lid down and over the lower lid.
4 If this does not rid the eye of the object, hold the eyelids apart and flush the eye gently with clean water.

WOUNDS AND EMBEDDED FOREIGN BODIES

Warning

- Do not attempt to examine the eye.
- Do not allow the sufferer to touch the eye.
- Do not attempt to remove any object embedded in any part of the eye.

Action

1 Lay the person down.
2 Place thick padding above and below the injured eye,

as shown below, then add a dressing. **Do not** allow the covering to press on the injured eye.

3 Seek medical aid urgently.

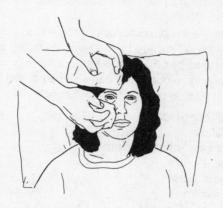

BLACK EYE

A severe blow to the eye area may cause BRUISES and internal bleeding.

Action

1 Check to see that the eye itself is not injured.

2 Apply an ice pack to the affected area (see SPRAINS AND DISLOCATIONS). **Do not** apply ice directly to the eye.

3 If the eye swells and closes, seek medical advice.

FAINTING

A person may lose consciousness if there is a temporary drop in the blood supply to the brain. Fainting may be caused by standing still for too long, especially in a hot, stuffy room or on a hot day. It can also be caused by lack of food, exhaustion or an emotional shock.

Signs and Symptoms
- unsteadiness
- pale, cold and clammy skin
- yawning
- slow, weak pulse
- blurred vision
- loss of consciousness

Warning
- A person who does regain consciousness quickly may be suffering from a more serious illness, such as STROKE or a heart condition (see HEART ATTACK and HEART FAILURE). Emergency first aid may be needed and medical help must be sought immediately.

Action
1 Lay the person down, with the feet raised.
2 Loosen any tight clothing and make sure there is adequate fresh air. Check that breathing and pulse are normal (see EMERGENCY TECHNIQUES).

3 Check for any injury or illness.
4 Encourage the person to rest for a while before moving, once consciousness has returned.

FISH HOOK INJURY

An embedded fish hook should be removed by a doctor but, if you are too far from medical help and it is a single-barbed hook just under the skin, you can remove it with care.

Action
1 **Do not** try to pull the hook out the way it went in. Push the hook out through the skin until the barb can be seen.

2 Cut off the barb.
3 Pull the shank of the hook out through the point of entry. (Alternatively, cut the shank off and pull the hook out by the barb).

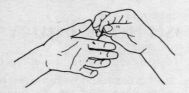

4 Apply a sterile pad to the wound and bandage firmly (see DRESSINGS, PADS AND BANDAGES).
5 A tetanus injection may need to be administered.

FRACTURES

A fracture is a broken or cracked bone. If the bone pierces the skin it is called a compound or open fracture. This fracture is very susceptible to infection and can result in considerable loss of blood.

If the skin has not been broken it is called a closed fracture (though there may be internal bleeding and damage).

In young children the bones, which are still flexible,

may not break completely. These incomplete breaks are called greenstick fractures.

If you suspect someone has a fracture, seek medical aid immediately.

Signs and Symptoms
- the sound or feel of a bone breaking
- intense pain around the break
- deformity of the limb or an inability to move it naturally
- tenderness when light pressure is applied
- swelling
- the sound of bone ends grating against each other

Warning
- Do not move the broken bone if possible.
- Do not shift the casualty, unless essential to safety, if there is a suspected back or neck fracture (see NECK AND SPINAL INJURIES) because the spinal cord can be damaged by movement.
- Do not administer any food or drink because a general anaesthetic may be needed.

Action
1 If there is an open wound, control BLEEDING and cover the wound with a sterile dressing; if the bone is protruding, use a ring pad (see DRESSINGS, PADS AND BANDAGES). Then apply a bandage, making sure it is not directly over the fracture.

2 Support the fractured limb in the most comfortable position. Raise and rest a fractured foot or ankle on pillows or folded blankets.

3 Immobilise the fractured limb, using a splint or sling (see SPLINTS and SLINGS for information on the splints and slings appropriate to different fractures). **Do not** attempt to straighten the fractured limb.

4 Check regularly that the bandages are not too tight, affecting circulation.

5 Watch for signs of SHOCK.

6 Seek medical aid immediately.

For the treatment of fractured ribs see CHEST INJURIES.

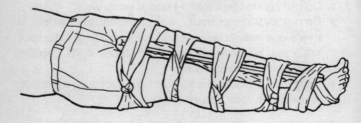

Fractured leg: pad well between the thighs and use a splint, if possible and the uninjured limb for support; secure the legs with bandages around the ankles and knees, also bandage above and below the fracture site and around the thighs, if help is likely to be delayed.

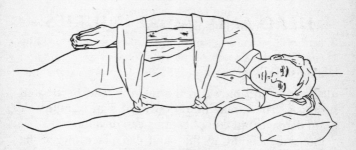

Fractured elbow if the arm is straight: lay the person down on the uninjured side, place the injured arm on a padded splint, along the side of the body, without bending the elbow, and secure the arm to the body (above and below the injury) with broad bandages tied on the uninjured side.

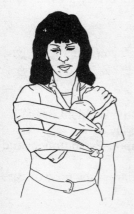

Fractured upper arm: apply a collar-and-cuff sling, pad the area between the body and the elbow and secure the arm to the body (above and below the injury) with broad bandages tied on the uninjured side.

HEAD AND FACIAL INJURIES

HEAD INJURY

All injuries and blows to the head should be treated seriously. There may be no outward sign of injury or brain damage, but complications can develop.

Internal bleeding in the skull can place increasing pressure on the brain and affect consciousness, breathing, pulse and blood pressure. In some cases loss of consciousness does not occur until some time after the accident.

Any casualty who has been even briefly unconscious must receive medical attention.

Signs and Symptoms
Note that some of the following symptoms and signs may not show immediately:
- headache and blurred vision
- nausea and vomiting
- loss of memory (especially of the accident itself)
- weakness on one side of the body
- confusion and abnormal responses to touch and commands
- bleeding or a flow of clear fluid from the nose or ears
- noisy breathing
- convulsions

- congested face
- wounds to the head or face
- one pupil larger than the other

Action

1 Treat the casualty as if unconscious: place him or her in the recovery position, check the airway, breathing and pulse and give AR or CPR if necessary (see EMERGENCY TECHNIQUES). **Do not** move the casualty, unless it is essential for safety, because there may be a spinal injury (see NECK AND SPINAL INJURIES). If you must move the casualty, support the head and neck and move gently (see MOVING A CASUALTY).

2 If the face is badly injured, keep the airway open with your fingers.

3 Control external BLEEDING. **Do not** apply pressure to the scalp if a fracture is suspected (see FRACTURES). If blood or fluid is coming from the ear, position the person as directed in EAR INJURIES. Lightly cover any EYE INJURIES with a clean dressing.

FRACTURED JAW

Signs and Symptoms

- swelling, pain or tenderness around the jaw
- misalignment of the jaw and teeth
- difficulty in closing the teeth
- drooling of saliva

Action

1 If the casualty is unconscious, place him or her in the recovery position, check the airway, breathing and pulse and begin AR or CPR if necessary (see EMERGENCY TECHNIQUES), supporting the jaw with your hand.
2 If the casualty is conscious and able to help, have him or her sit in the most comfortable position, supporting the jaw with a hand. **Do not** try to apply a jaw bandage.
3 Seek medical help immediately.

DISLOCATED JAW

Signs and Symptoms

As for a Fractured Jaw (see above).

Action

1 Remove any dentures.
2 Support the jaw.
3 Seek medical help.

See also CONCUSSION; TEETH INJURIES.

HEART ATTACK

A heart attack occurs when the blood supply to the heart is blocked by a blood clot in a coronary artery. Prompt first aid and immediate specialised medical attention could save a person's life.

Signs and Symptoms

- severe pain in the centre of the chest, which can spread to the arms (especially the left one), neck and jaw – the pain is sometimes mistaken for indigestion
- nausea and vomiting
- shortness of breath
- pale or blue, cold, clammy skin
- confusion or distress
- SHOCK
- collapse, leading to loss of pulse

Action

1 If the person is unconscious, place him or her in the recovery position, check the airway, breathing and pulse and begin AR or CPR if necessary (see EMERGENCY TECHNIQUES).

2 If the person is conscious, sit him or her up and loosen clothing.

3 Call for an ambulance immediately. **Make sure** you inform the service that the casualty has suffered a heart attack.

HEART FAILURE

The heart's ability to pump blood to the body may be impaired after a HEART ATTACK or because of heart disease or advanced age. Brain damage or death can quickly result from acute heart failure, so prompt first aid and medical attention are urgently required.

Signs and Symptoms
- severe shortage of breath
- chest pain
- noisy breathing
- rapid, weak pulse
- neck veins become swollen
- swollen legs and ankles
- blood-stained mucus coughed up
- bluish lips and extremities

Action
1 If the person is unconscious, place him or her in the recovery position, check the airway, breathing and pulse and begin AR or CPR if necessary (see EMERGENCY TECHNIQUES).
2 If the casualty is conscious, sit him or her up and loosen clothing.
3 Seek medical aid urgently.

HEAT EXHAUSTION AND HEAT STROKE

Heat exhaustion is the result of excessive loss of body fluid through perspiration.

Heat stroke is more unusual and more dangerous than heat exhaustion. It occurs when the body's heat-regulating mechanism fails completely. Early recognition and medical attention are essential.

Heat exhaustion and heat stroke are most likely to occur in hot, humid conditions, particularly if prolonged exercise is involved. The young and the old are the most susceptible because their bodies are the least efficient at regulating body temperature. **Never** leave a baby in a closed car on a hot day.

HEAT EXHAUSTION

Signs and Symptoms
- feeling of being hot and exhausted
- headache
- faintness and giddiness
- thirst
- nausea
- muscle cramps and weakness
- pale, cold, clammy skin

- heavy sweating
- rapid pulse and breathing
- lack of coordination
- confusion and irritability

Action

1 Move the sufferer to a cool place with fresh air.
2 Lay the person down. Loosen his or her clothing and remove any articles that are not needed.
3 Sponge the sufferer with cool water.
4 Encourage the person slowly to drink water, to which a small amount of salt is added.
5 Apply ice packs to cramped muscles (see SPRAINS AND DISLOCATIONS).
6 If the person does not recover quickly or vomits, seek medical aid immediately.

HEAT STROKE

Signs and Symptoms

- hot, flushed, dry skin
- headache
- dizziness
- rise in body TEMPERATURE to 40°C (104°F) or more
- rapid, pounding pulse
- nausea and vomiting
- confusion and irritability
- loss of consciousness

Action

1 If the casualty is unconscious, place him or her in the recovery position, check the airway, breathing and pulse and begin AR or CPR if necessary (see EMERGENCY TECHNIQUES).

2 Move the casualty to a cool place.

3 Loosen his or her clothing and remove any articles that are not needed.

4 Cool the casualty as quickly as possible: apply ice packs to the neck, groin and armpits (see SPRAINS AND DISLOCATIONS). Then wrap the person in a cool, wet sheet. Fan the casualty to increase the cooling process.

5 Check the casualty's temperature every 5 minutes. As soon as it is down to 38°C (100.4°F) and the skin feels cool, stop the cooling process.

6 Seek medical aid immediately.

7 When the casualty is conscious, give small, frequent sips of liquid as for Heat Exhaustion (see above).

NECK AND SPINAL INJURIES

Neck and spinal injuries must always be treated as serious. The casualty must be handled with the utmost care to prevent further damage that could result in permanent paralysis or even breathing and circulation failure.

Injury to the spine must always be suspected if the casualty is unconscious from a head injury (see HEAD AND FACIAL INJURIES).

Signs and Symptoms
- intense pain at or below the injury
- tenderness at the site of the injury
- tingling sensations in the hands or feet
- loss of movement or feeling at or below the injury

In cases of damage to the spinal cord, there may also be:

- loss of bowel or bladder control
- breathing difficulty
- SHOCK

Warning
- Never move a person with suspected spinal injuries unless essential to safety, for example, if unconscious. Leave moving a casualty to ambulance officers. If you must move the casualty, support the neck, head and spine (see MOVING A CASUALTY).
- Do not twist or bend an injured spine.

Action
1 If the casualty is unconscious, place him or her in the recovery position, carefully supporting the head and

neck with your hand, check the airway, breathing and pulse and begin AR or CPR if necessary (see EMERGENCY TECHNIQUES).

2 If the casualty is conscious, cover and keep him or her as still as possible. **Do not** attempt to raise the head or give anything to eat or drink. Loosen any tight clothing.

3 If the neck has been injured, and particularly if the person is trapped in an upright position, support the head and neck with your hands.

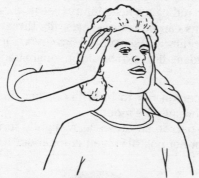

4 Seek medical aid urgently.

NOSEBLEED

A nosebleed can be caused by a heavy knock, blowing the nose too hard or high blood pressure. Sometimes it occurs for no apparent reason. Nosebleeds are quite common among children.

Warning
- Unconsciousness and a flow of pale fluid mixed with blood can indicate a head injury (see HEAD AND FACIAL INJURIES). This can be serious, even life-threatening, so emergency first aid (see EMERGENCY TECHNIQUES) may be required and medical aid should be sought immediately.

Action
1 Tell the person not to blow his or her nose and to breathe through the mouth.
2 Have the person sit down, lean slightly forward and hold his or her nostrils together for about 10 minutes.

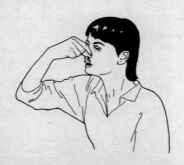

3 Loosen the clothing around the neck, chest and waist.
4 If the nose continues to bleed, repeat the procedure.
The person should not blow the nose for several hours
after bleeding has stopped.
5 If bleeding persists, seek medical advice.

OVER-EXPOSURE TO COLD

Prolonged exposure to cold conditions, particularly wet
and windy weather, or immersion in cold water can
cause the body's heat-regulating mechanism to fail, with
severe, even fatal results. Alcohol and drugs also decrease the functioning of the body's heat-regulating
mechanism.

Hypothermia is the extreme cooling of the body, often
caused by protracted immersion in cold water. After
the loss of the body's surface heat, there is a cooling of
deep tissues and organs.

As with over-exposure to heat, the young and the old
are the most susceptible because their bodies are the
least efficient at regulating body temperature. However,
even young, fit adults can be seriously affected if they are
exposed to extreme cold without adequate protection.

Prolonged exposure of the extremities to severe cold
can result in frostbite: the small blood vessels constrict

and cut the blood supply to the ears, nose, fingers or toes. In extreme cases, gangrene may develop and amputation may be necessary.

MILD TO MODERATE OVER-EXPOSURE

Signs and Symptoms
- shivering and a feeling of being cold
- extreme fatigue, drowsiness
- cramps
- blurred vision
- slowing of mental and physical alertness
- slurred speech and confusion
- stumbling, uncoordinated movement

Warning
- Do not attempt to warm the victim quickly by using an electric blanket or hot-water bottle or by placing the person close to a fire or heater.

Action
1 If the person is unconscious, place him or her in the recovery position, check the airway, breathing and pulse and begin AP or CPR if necessary (see EMERGENCY TECHNIQUES).
2 Move the person to a sheltered, dry spot. Replace wet clothes with warm, dry clothing, blankets or sleeping bag to prevent further heat loss. If it is available, use windproof material, such as aluminium foil or plastic,

for further protection. The body heat from another person is also a valuable aid: have someone, stripped to his or her underwear, share the blankets or sleeping bag with the sufferer.

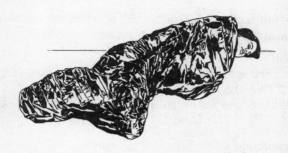

3 If the person is conscious, give him or her warm drinks. **Do not** give alcohol.
4 Seek medical advice.

EXTREME OVER-EXPOSURE (HYPOTHERMIA)

Signs and Symptoms
- skin is cold to the touch
- a baby's skin may look a healthy pink, but is cold to the touch
- slow and shallow breathing
- slow pulse
- a baby becomes quiet and refuses food
- unconsciousness, particularly of the old or infirm

Warning
- The warming process must be gradual: sudden heating could cause SHOCK.
- Do not place anyone suffering from hypothermia in a bath.
- Do not apply an electric blanket or hot-water bottle or warm the victim by a fire or heater.

Action
1 Proceed as for Mild to Moderate Over-exposure, steps 1–3 (see above).
2 Seek medical aid urgently and remain with the casualty until it is at hand.

FROSTBITE

Signs and Symptoms
- affected part is tingling or numb
- skin is waxy, white and firm to touch
- pain is not felt until the area becomes warm again
- blisters

Warning
- Do not rub or massage the affected part.
- Do not apply direct heat, cold water or snow.
- Do not give alcohol.

Action
1 Move the casualty to a warm, dry shelter if possible.
2 Warm the affected area slowly, using body heat. For

example, cup your hands around the affected part or have the sufferer put the part inside his or her clothing or under an armpit.

3 Cover any blisters with dry, sterile dressings.

4 Seek medical aid.

POISONING

Poisons can be swallowed, inhaled, absorbed or injected. Food, medicines and household and industrial products can all be poisonous.

Remember
- In many cases, accidental poisoning is avoidable (see FAMILY SAFETY).

Signs and Symptoms
Depending on the nature of the poison, signs and symptoms can include:

- pain, from the mouth to the abdomen
- nausea
- vomiting
- drowsiness
- faintness
- tight chest and difficulty breathing

- ringing ears
- headache
- odour of fumes
- sweating
- change of skin colour
- breath odour
- burns around and inside the mouth
- unconsciousness

For specific information on a poison contact your nearest hospital Accident and Emergency unit. (Check the telephone book and keep the number by the telephone in case of an emergency.)

General Action

1 If the casualty is unconscious, place him or her in the recovery position, check the airway, breathing and pulse and begin AR or CPR if necessary (see EMERGENCY TECHNIQUES). If AR or CPR is required, make sure you wipe any poisonous substance from the casualty's mouth first.

2 If the casualty is conscious, treat him or her according to the poison taken (see below). It is also important to establish what the drug or poison was because this may be of help in the medical treatment of the casualty.

3 Call for urgent medical aid.

CORROSIVE, PETROL-BASED OR UNKNOWN SUBSTANCES

Corrosives are substances, such as battery acid, dishwasher detergent, toilet cleaner and caustic soda, that burn tissues.

Warning
- Do not induce vomiting because it could cause further damage to tissues and the lungs.

Action
1 Wash the casualty's mouth and face clean of the substance. **Do not** give anything by mouth.
2 Seek medical aid urgently.

MEDICINAL AND GENERAL SUBSTANCES

General substances include plants, such as some mushrooms, and detergent.

Warning
- Do not attempt to induce vomiting if the casualty is unconscious or lying on his or her back.

Action
If your Accident and Emergency unit or doctor tells you to do so, give syrup of ipecacuanha, following the bottle's instructions, to induce vomiting. **Do not** use salted or soapy water to cause vomiting.

INHALED POISONS

Industrial gases, carbon monoxide (in car exhaust fumes) or the fumes from polyurethane foam can all cause poisoning.

Action

1 Take care not to breathe any toxic fumes or gas yourself. Cover your mouth and nose with a wet handkerchief. Ventilate the area thoroughly or move the casualty to fresh air if necessary.
2 If the casualty is unconscious, place him or her in the recovery position, check the airway, breathing and pulse and begin AR or CPR if necessary (see EMERGENCY TECHNIQUES).
3 Loosen any tight clothing.
4 Seek medical aid urgently.

ABSORBED POISONS

Toxic chemicals, such as pesticides, can be absorbed through the skin. It may take some time before the symptoms become evident. Check whether the casualty has been in contact with any poison from, for example, crop spraying.

Action

1 Get the casualty to remove the contaminated clothing and footwear. If you help, wear rubber gloves.

2 Wash the contaminated skin thoroughly with soap and water (and later wash the contaminated clothes separately from other articles).

3 Seek medical aid if any of the signs or symptoms of poisoning occur (see above). If you know the name of the chemical, let the doctor or hospital staff know.

4 If the casualty becomes unconscious, place him or her in the recovery position, check the airway, breathing and pulse and begin AR or CPR if necessary (see EMERGENCY TECHNIQUES).

See also BITES AND STINGS; VOMITING AND DIARRHOEA.

SHOCK

Clinical shock can occur when there is extreme pain, severe bleeding or heavy loss of fluid after, for example, major injury, vomiting, diarrhoea or burns.

Clinical shock is a serious, life-threatening condition. It occurs progressively, so watch closely for any signs, particularly deterioration in a casualty's condition after an accident or sudden illness.

Signs and Symptoms
- pale, cold, clammy skin
- weak, rapid pulse

- rapid breathing
- faintness, dizziness
- nausea
- thirst
- restlessness
- drowsiness and confusion, leading eventually to unconsciousness

Action

1 If the casualty is unconscious, place him or her in the recovery position, check the airway, breathing and pulse and begin AR or CPR if necessary (see EMERGENCY TECHNIQUES).

2 If the casualty is conscious, lay him or her down and, if possible, raise the legs (unless there are FRACTURES) and keep the head low to help the blood flow to the brain.

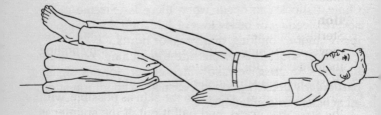

3 Because shock is brought on by major injury or illness you need to identify and treat its cause. (The casualty

may, for example, be BLEEDING heavily, have serious BURNS AND SCALDS or have suffered a HEART ATTACK.)

4 Seek medical aid urgently.

5 Loosen any tight clothing. Try to maintain the body temperature, but **do not** over-heat the casualty.

6 **Do not** give anything to eat or drink. If the casualty is thirsty, moisten the lips.

7 Monitor the airway, breathing and pulse regularly.

SPLINTERS

Even a tiny fragment of wood or glass or a thorn can cause an infection if not removed. Large splinters deeply embedded are best removed by a doctor.

Action

1 Sterilise splinter forceps, tweezers or splinter remover by burning the ends over a flame or by boiling them in water for 5 minutes.

2 Wash the area surrounding the splinter.

3 Grip the splinter, as close to the skin as possible, with the splinter forceps, and pull it out. If the splinter is too difficult to remove with forceps, use a splinter remover to expose the splinter then pull the splinter out.

4 Wash the wound with soapy water or mild antiseptic, dry it and, if necessary, cover it with an adhesive strip dressing.

5 If the wound becomes infected or swollen, seek medical advice.

SPRAINS AND DISLOCATIONS

When a joint is forced beyond its normal range of movement the ligaments that hold it together become sprained (that is, stretched or torn); the joint becomes dislocated if its bones are pushed out of contact with each other.

Sprains and dislocations are often associated with FRACTURES and have the same symptoms. If you are unsure, treat such an injury as a fracture and seek medical aid immediately.

The most common dislocations involve the shoulder, elbow, finger and jaw. Sprains often occur to ankles, but also affect wrists, elbows, knees, hips and shoulders.

SPRAINS

Signs and Symptoms
- pain and tenderness around the joint

- restricted movement of the joint
- swelling and bruising

Warning
- Do not move the joint if you suspect it is fractured.

Action

1 Remove clothing, shoes, etc. from the injured area. (Remember RICE: Rest, Ice, Compression, Elevation.)
2 Rest the joint in the most comfortable position and apply ice packs (see p. 120) to ease the pain and swelling.
3 Apply a compression bandage that extends well beyond the site (see DRESSINGS, PADS AND BANDAGES) and elevate the affected part.
4 Seek medical aid.

DISLOCATIONS

Signs and Symptoms
- intense pain
- deformity
- inability to move the joint
- swelling and bruising

Warning
- Do not move the joint if you suspect it is fractured.
- Do not attempt to push the joint bones back into position.

Action

1 Support and rest the joint in the most comfortable position.
2 Apply ice packs (see box).
3 Seek medical aid immediately.

For the treatment of a dislocated jaw see HEAD AND FACIAL INJURIES.

APPLYING ICE PACKS

1 Wrap ice in cloth. **Do not** apply ice directly to bare skin.
2 Apply ice packs for 30 minutes every 2 hours for the first 24 hours, then every 4 hours for a further 24 hours.

STRAINS

A strain results from a muscle or tendons being over-stretched during, for example, sport or a fall.

Signs and Symptoms

- sharp, sudden pain
- pain increases with movement

- tenderness around the muscle area
- loss of power

Action

1 Remove clothing, shoes, etc. from the affected area and place the person in a comfortable position, supporting the injured limb.
2 Remember RICE: Rest, Ice, Compression, Elevation as for SPRAINS AND DISLOCATIONS.
3 **Do not** massage the injured limb. Bandage it firmly (see DRESSINGS, PADS AND BANDAGES).
4 Getting the sufferer to exercise gently may help ease painful spasm.
5 Seek medical advice if the pain persists.

STROKE

Stroke refers to the brain damage caused by a blocked or ruptured artery in the brain. Elderly people with high blood pressure are particularly susceptible to stroke.

Signs and Symptoms
- weakness or paralysis on one side of the body
- confusion
- unconsciousness

- severe headache
- difficulty swallowing
- pounding pulse
- red face
- difficulty speaking
- seizures, sometimes

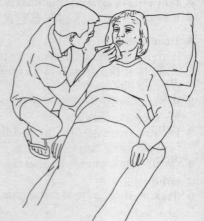

Action

1 If the casualty is unconscious, place him or her in the recovery position, check the airway, breathing and pulse and begin AR or CPR if necessary (see EMERGENCY TECHNIQUES).

2 Seek medical aid urgently.

3 If the casualty is conscious, prop him or her on pillows and loosen any tight clothing. Keep the person warm and wipe away any dribbled secretions.

SUNBURN

Over-exposure to strong sun, particularly in the middle of the day, can cause redness, inflammation, swelling and blistered skin, which will eventually dry out and flake off. In the long term over-exposure can lead to freckling, blotchy skin and even skin cancer. Children are especially vulnerable and need maximum protection.

Remember
- The best cure is prevention. Stay out of the sun in the heat of the day, wear adequate clothing, a hat and a total sun-block lotion.

Action
1 Move the person inside or into the shade.
2 Reduce the pain with a cool shower, bath or compress to the affected part, but **do not** chill the person. Be careful not to break any blisters.
3 Give plenty of cool fluids.
4 The sufferer should cover the sunburn if going out in the sun.
5 Seek medical aid if a person with blisters or a young child is involved.

See also HEAT EXHAUSTION AND HEAT STROKE.

SWALLOWED OBJECTS

Swallowed objects are a common occurrence, especially with young children. Very small, smooth objects may not be a problem, but sharp, jagged objects, such as bones, nails or glass, can be dangerous.

Always check children's and babies' toys to make sure there are no loose, small or sharp parts that could easily be swallowed.

Action
1 **Do not** give anything to eat or drink.
2 Take the child to hospital immediately.

See also CHOKING.

TEETH INJURIES

A tooth that has been knocked out of the mouth can be saved if you act quickly. Baby or first teeth, however, should not be replaced. Anyone who has damaged his or her teeth should see a dentist as soon as possible.

Action

1 Clean the tooth that has been knocked out, by having the casualty suck it. If this is not possible, use saliva or milk that has not been warmed. If there is no other option, wash the tooth under tap water.

2 Place the tooth in its original socket and hold it there for 2 minutes.

3 Mould a piece of aluminium foil over it and the two teeth on either side to form a temporary splint. The casualty should bite down to keep this in place.

4 If the tooth cannot be replaced in the mouth immediately, keep it moist in saliva or milk.

5 Seek dental aid immediately.

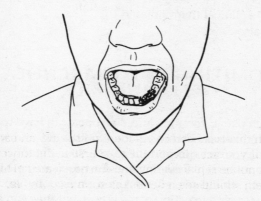

TEMPERATURE

The body's temperature can vary during the day and can be affected by hot weather, physical exertion or hot food or drink; the normal range is 36°C (96.8°F) to 37°C (98.6°F).

Lowered or raised temperature can indicate illness or major injury. For example, low temperature can indicate SHOCK, heavy BLEEDING or hypothermia (see OVER-EXPOSURE TO COLD); high temperature can indicate severe infection or heat stroke (see HEAT EXHAUSTION AND HEAT STROKE).

A mercury thermometer is the most common and accurate clinical thermometer.

VOMITING AND DIARRHOEA

Stomach pains, vomiting and diarrhoea can have many different causes, including food poisoning and viral infections, so it is important to see your doctor if the symptoms persist. Vomiting and diarrhoea are common in young children and are often caused by gastro-enteritis, a viral infection of the bowel, but they can also be caused by other infections.

TAKING THE TEMPERATURE

1 Wash and dry the thermometer, then shake the mercury column down until the reading is below 36°C (96.8°F).

2 Place the thermometer bulb under the tongue, under the arm or in the groin. Leave it there for 3 minutes before taking the reading. Babies and small children should have their temperature taken under the arm because they cannot hold the thermometer properly in their mouth and may also bite it. Temperature taken in this way reads 0.5°C less than in the mouth. Thus an armpit temperature of 37°C (98.6°F) indicates a fever.

Food poisoning often results from eating food contaminated by bacteria. Bacteria can breed in foods, such as fish, chicken, ham and dairy products, that are not properly handled. Food should always be well cooked and eaten immediately or refrigerated as soon as it is bought. If food is reheated always bring it to boiling point. Food poisoning can also result from naturally occurring toxins in some plants and fish (see POISONING).

Vomiting and diarrhoea can cause dehydration – loss of the fluids required for the normal functioning of the body – particularly in babies and small children, so it is important that sufferers drink lots of fluid.

GASTROENTERITIS IN BABIES AND YOUNG CHILDREN

Signs and Symptoms

In addition to vomiting and the passing of frequent watery stools there may be the following signs and symptoms of dehydration:

- decrease in urine passed or number of wet nappies
- tiredness and listlessness
- refusal of food and drink
- dry mouth and tongue
- pale and thin appearance
- sunken-looking eyes
- cold hands and feet
- child is difficult to wake

Action

1 Stop solid food and cow's milk (but continue breast milk if the child is breast fed) and give rehydration fluid to drink: 1 cup (150–200 ml) every time the child vomits or passes a watery stool. If vomiting is frequent, give smaller amounts more often: 50 ml every 15 minutes. Suitable rehydration fluids are Dioralyte or Rehidrat, which can be bought at a chemist; they should be made up carefully according to the instruc-

tions on the container. You can also give: sugar (1 level teaspoon) plus a small pinch of salt per 120 ml water. If nothing else is available, use cordial that is not low calorie (1 part to 6 parts water), natural fruit juice (1 part to 4 parts water) or lemonade that is not low calorie (1 part to 4 parts water). **Remember** to dilute these liquids as described here; if they are given undiluted they may make the diarrhoea worse. **Do not** stop solid food and milk for more than 24 hours.

2 After the first 24 hours continue to give rehydration fluid between meals, but reintroduce solid food and cow's milk. Start with cooked vegetables and cereals, including bread, then add dairy products, eggs and meat.

3 Seek medical aid if: the child has a lot of diarrhoea (8–10 watery stools or 2–3 very large stools a day); vomiting persists and little fluid is kept down; there are signs of dehydration; the child develops severe stomach pain.

OTHER TITLES IN THE SERIES